Health Evidence Network synthesis report **57**

What is the evidence on existing policies and linked activities and their effectiveness for improving health literacy at national, regional and organizational levels in the WHO European Region?

Gillian Rowlands | Siân Russell | Amy O'Donnell | Eileen Kaner | Anita Trezona
Jany Rademakers | Don Nutbeam

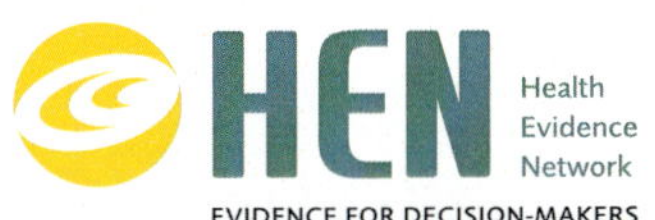

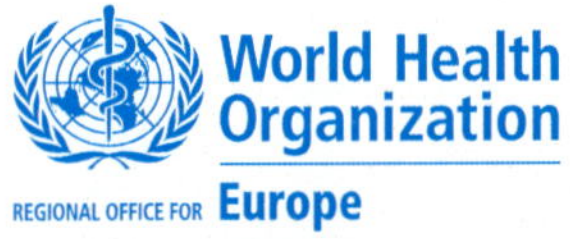

Abstract

Health literacy is gaining increasing attention as a means of promoting health. This evidence synthesis describes health literacy policies in the WHO European Region: their distribution, organizational levels, antecedents, actors, activities and outcomes, along with the factors influencing their effectiveness. Evidence was obtained by a scoping review of academic literature in English, Dutch and German and of grey literature in English, Dutch, German and Italian, supported by a Region-wide expert enquiry. Emerging findings were presented to representatives from 19 Member States of the Region to check for accuracy and omissions. The report highlights much good health literacy policy-related activity, mostly in the health and education sectors, and proposes areas for future development. Policy considerations to facilitate the sharing of good health literacy policy practice, the development of policy aims and activities across all societal areas, and the development of robust health literacy metrics to identify the need for and monitor effectiveness are presented.

Keywords

HEALTH LITERACY; PATIENT EDUCATION AS TOPIC; CONSUMER HEALTH INFORMATION; HEALTH EDUCATION; HEALTH PROMOTION; EUROPE

Suggested citation

Rowlands G, Russell S, O'Donnell A, Kaner E, Trezona A, Rademakers J et al. What is the evidence on existing policies and linked activities and their effectiveness for improving health literacy at national, regional and organizational levels in the WHO European Region? Copenhagen: WHO Regional Office for Europe; 2018 (Health Evidence Network (HEN) synthesis report 57).

Address requests about publications of the WHO Regional Office for Europe to:
Publications
WHO Regional Office for Europe
UN City, Marmorvej 51
DK-2100 Copenhagen Ø, Denmark
Alternatively, complete an online request form for documentation, health information, or for permission to quote or translate, on the Regional Office website (http://www.euro.who.int/pubrequest).

ISSN 2227-4316
ISBN 978 92 890 5319 8

© World Health Organization 2018

All rights reserved. The Regional Office for Europe of the World Health Organization welcomes requests for permission to reproduce or translate its publications, in part or in full.

The designations employed and the presentation of the material in this publication do not imply the expression of any opinion whatsoever on the part of the World Health Organization concerning the legal status of any country, territory, city or area or of its authorities, or concerning the delimitation of its frontiers or boundaries. Dotted lines on maps represent approximate border lines for which there may not yet be full agreement.

The mention of specific companies or of certain manufacturers' products does not imply that they are endorsed or recommended by the World Health Organization in preference to others of a similar nature that are not mentioned. Errors and omissions excepted, the names of proprietary products are distinguished by initial capital letters.

All reasonable precautions have been taken by the World Health Organization to verify the information contained in this publication. However, the published material is being distributed without warranty of any kind, either express or implied. The responsibility for the interpretation and use of the material lies with the reader. In no event shall the World Health Organization be liable for damages arising from its use. The views expressed by authors, editors, or expert groups do not necessarily represent the decisions or the stated policy of the World Health Organization.

CONTENTS

ABBREVIATIONS

EU	European Union
MiMi	With Migrants for Migrants – Intercultural Health in Germany (programme)

CONTRIBUTORS

This report has been produced with the financial assistance of the Federal Office for Public Health, Switzerland. The views expressed herein can in no way be taken to reflect the official opinion of the Federal Office for Public Health, Switzerland.

Authors

Gillian Rowlands
Professor of Primary Care, Institute of Health and Society, Newcastle University, United Kingdom

Siân Russell
Research Associate, Institute of Health and Society, Newcastle University, United Kingdom

Amy O'Donnell
NIHR School for Primary Care Research Postdoctoral Fellow, Institute of Health and Society, Newcastle University, United Kingdom

Eileen Kaner
Professor of Public Health, Institute of Health and Society, Newcastle University, United Kingdom

Anita Trezona
Health Literacy Policy Researcher, Melbourne, Australia

Jany Rademakers
Head of Research Department, NIVEL, Netherlands Institute for Health Services Research in Utrecht and Professor of Health Literacy and Patient Participation, CAPHRI, Department of General Practice, Maastricht University, Maastricht, the Netherlands

Don Nutbeam
Professor of Public Health, School of Public Health, University of Sydney, Australia

External peer reviewers

Jürgen M. Pelikan
Emeritus Professor of Sociology, University of Vienna, and Director, Competence Center Health Promotion in Hospitals and Health Care, Gesundheit Österreich GmbH, Vienna, Austria

Stephan Van den Broucke
Professor of Public Health Psychology, Institut de Recherche en Sciences Psychologiques, Faculté de Psychologie et des Sciences de l'Education, Université Catholique de Louvain, Louvain-la-Neuve, Belgium

Collaborators

Paloma Amil-Bujan (Health Ministry, Barcelona, Spain), Fleur Braddick (Health Ministry, Barcelona, Spain), Janine Bröder (Bielefeld University, Germany), Xavier Debussche (Centre Hospitalier Universitaire de La Réunion, Saint-Denis Réunion, France), Oriol Garcia-Codina (Health Ministry, Barcelona, Spain), Karin Gasser (Federal Office of Public Health, Switzerland), Concepció González-Mestre (Health Ministry, Barcelona, Spain), Sandra Husbands (Abertawe Bro Morgannwg University Health Board, Port Talbot, Wales), Diane Levin-Zamir (Clalit Health Services & School of Public Health, University of Haifa, Israel), Christos Lionis (University of Crete, Greece), Maria Lopatina (Ministry of Health, Russian Federation), Alba Martínez García (Alicante University, Spain), Anne McCusker (Belfast Healthy Cities, Belfast, United Kingdom), Orkan Okan (Bielefeld University, Germany), Mike Oliver (Stoke-on-Trent City Council, United Kingdom), Leena Paakkari (University of Jyväskylä, Finland), Nicola Pavese (Newcastle University, Newcastle upon Tyne, United Kingdom), Elena Petelos (University of Crete, Greece), Sebastian Potthoff (Newcastle University, Newcastle upon Tyne, United Kingdom), Luis A. Saboga-Nunes (Universidade NOVA de Lisboa, Portugal), Doris Schaeffer (Bielefeld University, Germany), Falko Sniehotta (Newcastle University, Newcastle upon Tyne, United Kingdom), Athanassios Vozikis (University of Piraeus, Greece), Heide Weishaar (Hertie School of Governance, Berlin, Germany).

Editorial team, WHO Regional Office for Europe

Division of Noncommunicable Diseases and Promoting Health through the Life-course

Martin Weber
Programme Manager, Child and Adolescent Health

Division of Information, Evidence, Research and Innovation

Ryoko Takahashi
Technical Officer, Knowledge Management, Evidence and Research for Policy-making Unit

Health Evidence Network (HEN) editorial team

Claudia Stein, Director
Tanja Kuchenmüller, a.i. Editor in Chief
Ryoko Takahashi, Series Editor
Krista Kruja, Consultant
Andrew Booth, Support to the HEN Secretariat
Ashley Craig, Technical Editor

The HEN Secretariat is part of the Division of Information, Evidence, Research and Innovation at the WHO Regional Office for Europe. HEN synthesis reports are commissioned works that are subjected to international peer review, and the contents are the responsibility of the authors. They do not necessarily reflect the official policies of the Regional Office.

SUMMARY

The issue

Health literacy is the capacity of individuals, families and communities to make sound health decisions in the context of everyday life: at home and the workplace; and in the community, marketplace, health care system and political arena. Increasing health literacy is a critical empowerment strategy to increase people's control over their health through improving their ability to seek out health information, express themselves on health issues and take responsibility for their health. Low health literacy is associated with poorer health, more illness and health inequalities, and it is likely to be associated with less cost-effective health systems. Addressing the issue of low health literacy, therefore, has the potential to increase health, health equity and health system effectiveness through building citizens' capacities for health.

The synthesis question

The objective of this report is to address the question "What is the evidence on existing policies and linked activities and their effectiveness for improving health literacy at national, regional and organizational levels in the WHO European Region?"

Types of evidence

The report identified policies and other relevant documents through an evidence review of peer-reviewed and grey literature, supplemented by an enquiry of experts in health, health literacy and policy in the Region and by health literacy policies included in the most recent peer-reviewed document on health literacy activities published in the Region (European Union (EU) countries only: HEALIT4EU). Further efforts to identify policies from countries of the Commonwealth of Independent States were unfruitful.

Results

This synthesis identified 46 existing and/or developing health literacy policies at international (for three Member States), national[1] and local levels in 19 of the 53 Member States of the Region (36%). Five policies were under development, 30 were currently active and 11 were time limited, with no evidence of a follow-on policy.

1 The national level includes policies for which both the strategy and the funding are devolved from the Member State to the individual country or semiautonomous region.

Policies were examined to (i) describe the policy stages; and (ii) analyse the components (antecedents, actors, activities and beneficiaries) and activities using a new framework, the Health Literacy Policy Model. A wide range of activities was identified at international, national and local levels. Baseline health literacy data are not available in all Member States. Evidence is emerging of successful activities to build health literacy at the individual and community levels, particularly in the areas of health and education, with some activities in the workplace. More activities are focused on building skills in individuals than in communities. Many policies have complementary areas of focus, where sharing of knowledge and resources could be beneficial. There is currently little evidence of activities and effectiveness in the areas of the lived environment, the media and digital/e-health literacy, although some of this information may be provided when evaluations of current projects are published. A low rate of policy identification through searching the peer-reviewed literature may reflect lack of engagement in policy evaluation by the academic community. Finally, policy-makers should be made aware of the facilitators of successful health literacy policy implementation, such as intersectoral working, political leadership and overcoming cultural barriers, and ensure that potential barriers to success, such as lack of evidence of the health, social and economic benefits of the policies, are addressed through rigorous evaluation. The economic effect of health literacy policy is an important area for development, as this evidence synthesis did not identify any evaluation of economic effects arising from the policies.

Policy considerations

Based on this evidence synthesis, the following policy considerations are proposed:

- consider the existing policies and related activities gathered in this review to develop or enhance health literacy policies and related activities to benefit citizens, patients and communities;
- broaden the range of areas of activity required for holistic health literacy policies to include the lived environment, the workplace, the media and digital/e-health, at all societal levels – individual, community, organization and system (legislative);
- strengthen the evidence base for health literacy at all societal levels to ensure that policies address needs specific to the national or local context;
- incorporate robust qualitative and quantitative evaluations into health literacy policies and interventions – quantitative methods could include pre- and post-activity health literacy evaluations of evidence of health, social and economic effects at all levels; and

- incorporate facilitators of successful implementation, such as intersectoral working, political leadership and strategies to overcome cultural barriers, into health literacy policy.

Member States would benefit from adopting such comprehensive frameworks and using metrics to design effective policies that support the development of a health-literate Europe.

1. INTRODUCTION

1.1 Background

The WHO European Region comprises 53 Member States with a combined population of 894 million (1). Member States have a wide range of cultures and economies: four are classified as having a lower-middle income, five as having an upper-middle income and 44 as having a high income (2). The Region is served by the WHO Regional Office for Europe, one of WHO's six regional offices around the world.

According to Sørensen et al., "health literacy is linked to literacy and entails people's knowledge, motivation and competences to access, understand, appraise and apply health information in order to make judgements and take decisions in everyday life concerning healthcare, disease prevention and health promotion to maintain or improve quality of life during the life course" (3). Suboptimal health literacy across the European Region is associated with illness and its economic costs. The prevalence of low (i.e. problematic and inadequate) health literacy was highlighted in the 2011 European health literacy survey of eight European Member States: Austria, Bulgaria, Germany (North Rhine-Westphalia), Greece, Ireland, the Netherlands, Poland and Spain (4). Although the prevalence of low health literacy varied considerably across Member States, when taken together, the health literacy of 47.6% of the adult population was below the recommended level. In all, 12.4% of the adult population had the lowest level of health literacy and would thus be expected to experience severe difficulties. The reasons underlying variations between countries are complex but likely to include factors such as variation in general literacy and numeracy levels, cultural differences and variations in the complexity of health systems (5). The 2011 European health literacy survey confirmed the findings of previous research outside Europe showing that low health literacy is linked to lower self-rated health and higher rates of chronic (i.e. long-term) health conditions (4,6). It also confirmed that a social gradient in health literacy exists: those already at an increased risk of poor health through age, socioeconomic deprivation and membership of minority ethnic groups were also more likely to have lower health literacy (4).

There are challenges for health systems to produce optimal outcomes for both patients and tax-payers: patients are experiencing poorer health and more illness than they might otherwise, and health services are struggling to be cost-effective in the face of increasing demands from an ageing population with rising levels of chronic disease (7). Improving health literacy, with a focus on building the health capacities of citizens and on increasing the responsiveness and skills of the health system and practitioners, is gaining increasing traction as a strategy to address these problems. It is a key component of Health 2020, the European health policy framework that supports action across government and society to improve the health and well-being of populations, reduce health inequities, strengthen public health and ensure people-centred health systems that are universal, equitable, sustainable and of high quality (8). However, evidence on the financial effects of health literacy on health service costs is limited. In the United States of America and Europe, low health literacy is associated with greater health care costs (9,10). Moreover, a Belgian study showed that low health literacy is associated with greater use of health care services, particularly the more specialized services (10).

Increasing recognition of the importance of health literacy has led to several key political statements. At the global level, the WHO 2017 Shanghai Declaration on promoting health in the 2030 Agenda for Sustainable Development (11) states that:

> *Health literacy empowers individual citizens and enables their engagement in collective health promotion action. A high health literacy of decision-makers and investors supports their commitment to health impact, co-benefits and effective action on the determinants of health. Health literacy is founded on inclusive and equitable access to quality education and lifelong learning. It must be an integral part of the skills, and competencies developed over a lifetime, first and foremost through the school curriculum.*

In the Shanghai Declaration, WHO made commitments to investing in health literacy as a critical determinant of health; developing, implementing and monitoring intersectoral national and local strategies for strengthening health literacy in all populations and in educational settings; increasing citizens' control of their own health and its determinants through harnessing the potential of digital technology; and ensuring that consumer environments support healthy choices through pricing policies, transparent information and clear labelling. Within the European Region, the European Parliament has endorsed the report Accelerating the health literacy agenda in Europe (12) and has published a policy brief highlighting the importance of health literacy through the life-course and the benefits of focusing health literacy interventions on children and young people (13). Health literacy is a key component of the 2013 Vilnius Declaration on sustainable health systems for inclusive growth (14) and the 2015 Riga roadmap (15). The 2015 Minsk Declaration emphasizes the importance of building skills through the life-course (from early years, through school years and into adulthood) (16), while the 2016 Paris Declaration highlights the importance of intersectoral and cross-government policies to promote health literacy, and hence health and well-being, in preschool and school children (17). Finally, the 2017 Healthy Cities Pécs Declaration highlights the roles of cities and communities as enablers of health and well-being for all (18). Guidelines for action have been published by the WHO Regional Office for Europe (19) and by Member States (20,21). The WHO Regional Office for Europe guidelines, Health literacy: the solid facts, highlight that health literacy involves more than just health systems and education systems: it exists "in the context of everyday life: at home, in the community, at the workplace, in the health care system, the marketplace and the political arena" (19,22), as well as, increasingly, the media, social media and digital health (19).

Health literacy is a rapidly expanding field. Previous reviews of health literacy policy include one by the United States Institute of Medicine (23) and another from the EU, the Study on sound evidence for a better understanding of health literacy in the EU (HEALIT4EU project) (5). This evidence synthesis differs from these in its perspective (European vs American), geographical scope (the whole of the WHO European Region vs the EU) and emphasis on synthesis of the findings. The aim was to identify and collate findings from policies and related activities in the Region; describe their effectiveness for improving health literacy at Regional, Member State and organizational levels; and propose policy considerations to enable all European citizens to enjoy the benefits of improved health literacy.

1.2 Methodology

As the definitions and concepts of health literacy are broad (3), overlapping with those of health promotion and health education (24), this scoping review considered only evidence in health policies that (i) met an adapted WHO definition (25) of "decisions, plans, and actions that are undertaken to achieve specific health literacy goals within a society" and (ii) included the term health literacy (or its equivalent in the national language). A search of peer-reviewed literature on policies and policy barriers, facilitators and effectiveness in English, Dutch and German, and of policies in the grey literature in English, Catalan, Dutch, French, German, Italian, Russian and Spanish, along with those identified through an expert enquiry and in the most recent peer-reviewed report, the 2013 HEALIT4EU study (5), was carried out between 9 October 2017 and 20 January 2018. Efforts were also made to identify policies from countries of the Commonwealth of Independent States.

A total of 15300 peer-reviewed articles were found after removal of duplicates and screening and 12 full-text articles were assessed for eligibility, resulting in the identification of four policy-related activities (26–29) linked with four policies (30–33) and three papers exploring barriers and facilitators to successful policy implementation (34–36). In addition, 15 policies were identified in the grey literature, along with 26 from the expert enquiry and seven from the HEALIT4EU study. After removal of duplicates, a total of 46 health literacy policies (30–33,37–78) and three articles on policy barriers/facilitators/effectiveness were identified (34–36).

Preliminary findings were presented to the WHO European Health Information Initiative Action Network on Measuring Health Literacy, involving 19 Member States of the Region, for quality checking and identification of any missed policies.

Fig. 1 shows the geographical distribution of documents from Member States of the European Region used in this review.

Annex 1 has full details of the methodology.

Fig. 1. Geographical distribution of Member States in which policies were identified

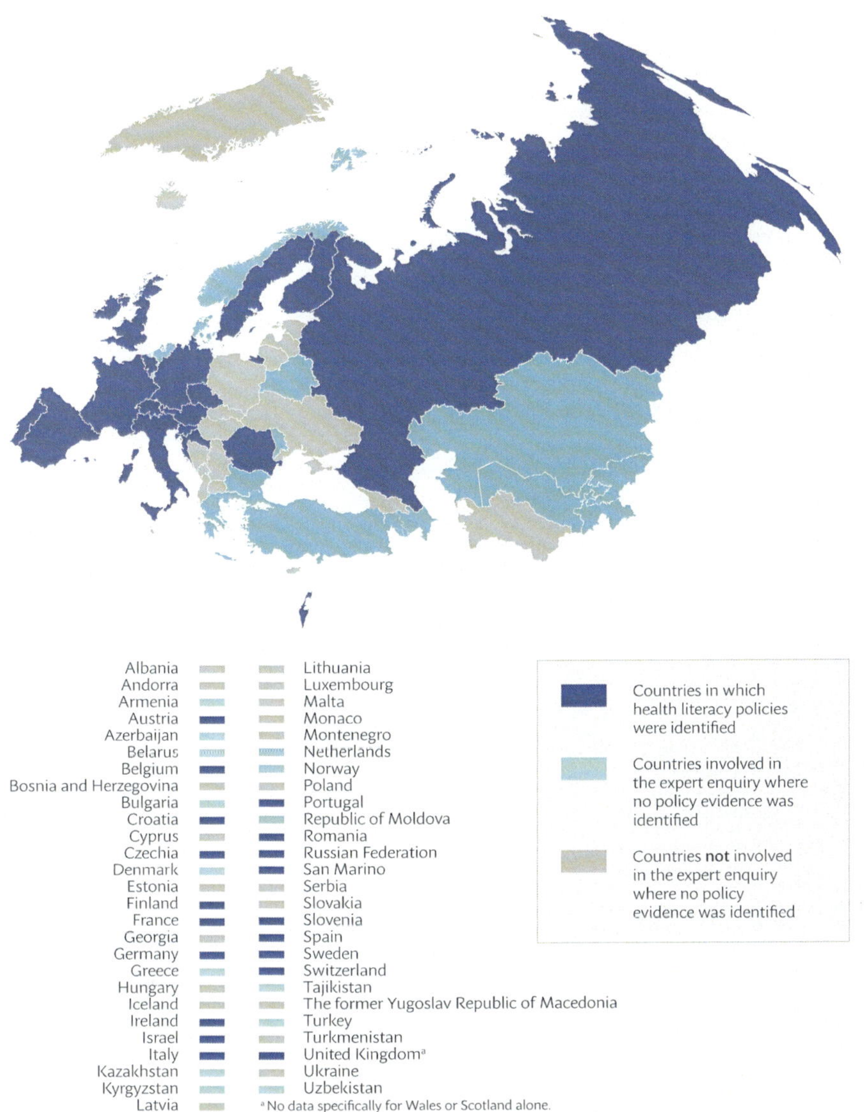

2. RESULTS

2.1 Overview of health literacy policies in the WHO European Region

A total of 19 Member States had recognized low health literacy as an issue and were either in the process of developing, or had developed, policy to address it: Austria, Belgium, Croatia, Czechia, Finland, France, Germany, Ireland, Israel, Italy, Portugal, Romania, the Russian Federation, San Marino, Slovenia, Spain, Sweden, Switzerland and the United Kingdom.

The governance level at which the policy had been developed was subdivided into four levels: regional (i.e. WHO European Region level), national (i.e. Member State level or country or administrative region in Member States where health policy and funding are devolved, e.g. Italy, Spain and the United Kingdom) and local (administrative regions, city or nongovernmental organization). Policies that involved more than one Member State but were not regional were classified as international. No regional policies were identified, although one (the MiMi programme (50)) was international, having started in Germany and spread to Austria and Switzerland. Of the remaining 45 policies, 37 were national and eight were local.

Next, policy stages were stratified by governance level according to an amended version of the Stages Model (79) as: under development (problem definition and agenda-setting); active (implementation and evaluation); or time limited with no evidence of a replacement policy. Five policies were under development: these were all national (38,46,60,63,65). A total of 30 policies were active: one was international (50), 23 were national (32,33,37,41–43,47–49,51,54–57,59,62,66–68,70,73,76,77) and six were local (31,40,53,71,74,78). Eleven policies were time limited and had ended: these were all national (30,39,44,45,52,58,61,64,69,72,75).

2.2 Policy analysis

Information was available for 43 of the 46 policies identified: the other three policies (from Belgium (38), Russia (63) and Slovenia (65)) were under development and further information was not available.

Policies and their components were assessed using criteria adapted from Cheung et al. (80) as: antecedents (the reasons underlying the policy); actors (people working or living in the sectors, organizations, professions and societal groups that need to be engaged for the policy to be effective); activities (actions to be undertaken to achieve the policy aims, including the development of publically accessible health literacy portals); whether or not evaluation was planned, and if planned whether it had taken place; and evidence of effectiveness. Actors were subclassified as either beneficiaries or implementers. The match between stated antecedents and available health literacy data was investigated.

The health literacy policies focused on a number of interlinked sectors and societal levels (19) and included a wide range of activities. To analyse activities directly linked to the identified policies, the Health Literacy Policy Model (including four societal levels and six vectors) was developed iteratively during evidence collation and synthesis (Fig. 2). The term vector was used to describe the various means by which health literacy could be developed: health, education through the life-course, the lived environment, employment, media, and digital/ e-health literacy (i.e. the ability to seek, find, understand and appraise health information from electronic sources and apply the knowledge gained to addressing or solving a health problem (81)).

Evidence synthesized from all policies is available on request.[2]

Fig. 2. The Health Literacy Policy Model

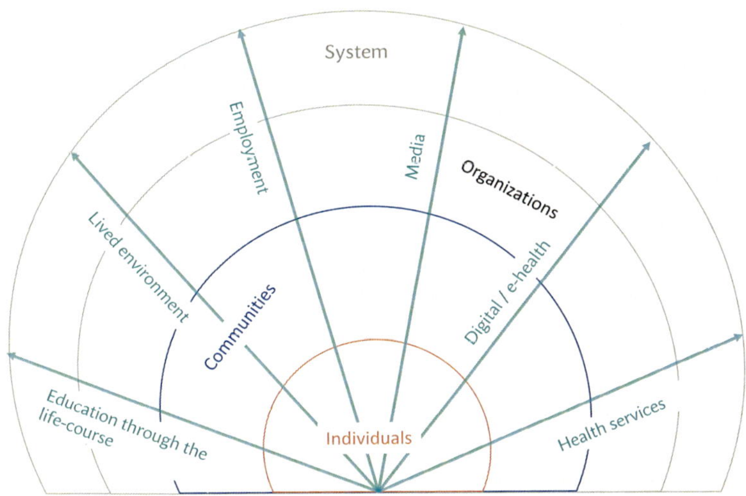

2 Details of all policies are available on request from euhen@who.int (Table 1. Policy details).

2.2.1 Policy antecedents

The 43 policies included in the analysis included 102 antecedents. These were mapped to societal levels in the Health Literacy Policy Model.

Individual level. A total of 47 antecedents mapped to this level, with most relating to health: low health literacy of individuals (e.g. patients, citizens, employees; *n* = 23) (37,41,44,46–48,50,51,54,55,57,58,62,64,66,67,69–71,73–75,78); high numbers of people with preventable disease (*n* = 9) (32,41,43,46,56,57,66,68,77); high numbers of people with low health (*n* = 7) (30,41,51,56,59,67,77); low e-health literacy (*n* = 3) (41,53,57); and high numbers of individuals with risky health behaviours (*n* = 4) (59,62,68,78). One antecedent was a lack of wider life skills (employability) in individuals (30).

Community level. Eight antecedents mapped to this level. All except one of these referred to vulnerable populations, such as migrants and refugees (33,50,54,69) (one policy had two antecedents (50)) and socioeconomically excluded and vulnerable groups (30,73). The remaining policy referred to communities in a more general sense (78).

Organization level. Forty antecedents from 36 policies mapped to this level; most of these related to health organizations. Fifteen policies had one or more antecedents related to low organizational awareness and responsiveness to health literacy (37,40,41,46,49,50,52,53,55,56,66,69,71,76,78), 10 policies mentioned low levels of health literacy competencies in the health workforce (37,40,41,45,46,54,55,70,75,78) and eight cited the complexity of current health information (40,45,47,55,56,58,68,76). One policy cited the lack of a national health literacy resource (75); one cited low health literacy in the media (56) and another cited low health literacy in (non-health) public sector organizations (71).

System level. Seven antecedents mapped to this level: two of these were linked to environmental safety (43,51), four to societal health inequalities (37,43,68,77) and one to a lack of health literacy awareness at the policy level (76).

Comparison revealed a mismatch between antecedents and the availability of relevant data. Although low health literacy of individuals was cited 23 times, the national health literacy level was known in only 15 cases. Similarly, nine policies linked health literacy to health inequalities between individuals or groups or at a societal level (although health literacy levels were known in only five of the countries) and another nine to chronic disease (although health literacy levels were known in four of the countries). Other antecedents supported by few quantitative data were low health literacy competencies in health workers and health material being too complex. No available baseline quantitative data were found for two antecedents: low levels of health literacy responsiveness in health organizations (mentioned in 15 policies) and low e-health literacy (mentioned in three policies).

2.2.2 Policy actors

Actors are defined as the people working or living in the sectors, organizations, professions and societal groups affected by a specific policy. They can be either beneficiaries of or implementers of policy activities.

Beneficiaries. The analysed policies included beneficiaries at both the individual and community levels. Those at the individual level included patients (31,32,37,40,43,45–47,51–53,55–58,66–68,70,75,76,78), citizens (37,43,45,47–49,51–57,62,64,66–68,70,72–74,78), learners (preschool (71), school students (42,51,59) and adults (44,45,70,71,74)), employees (40,44,72) and prisoners (72). At the community level, most beneficiaries were people in vulnerable groups such as children in socioeconomically deprived families (42,51,59), older people (57), migrant groups (33,54,69), pregnant women (62) and socioeconomically excluded and vulnerable groups (30,73). Wider communities were cited in one policy (78). Families were cited as beneficiaries in five policies (37,59,62,71,73).

Implementers. As implementers generally work for organizations and public bodies, most mapped to the organization level in the Health Literacy Policy Model. Most implementers work in organizations within the public sector, such as those in the health (31,32,37,40,41,43,45–47,51–53,55–57,66–68,70,75,76,78) and education (30,42,44,45,48–51,59,64,70–74) sectors, as well as social services, the fire service, the police or prison service (30,70–72). Some implementers work for health and/or social insurance organizations (37,47,49), nongovernment organizations (such as community liaison groups, charities and some health providers (31,33,47,49,52,54,57,62,73)) and trade unions (48). Finally, three policies cited people working for commercial organizations (48,49,56) and two cited workers from research organizations (43,77). People working at the system level (i.e. in national or local government) were cited in eight policies (30,46,49,51,68,73,77); no policies cited people working at the international or regional levels.

Beneficiaries and implementers were mapped to the Health Literacy Policy Model (Fig. 3). Beneficiaries mapped to the individual and community levels, with most

Fig. 3. Numbers of beneficiaries and implementers mapped to the four levels of the Health Literacy Policy Model

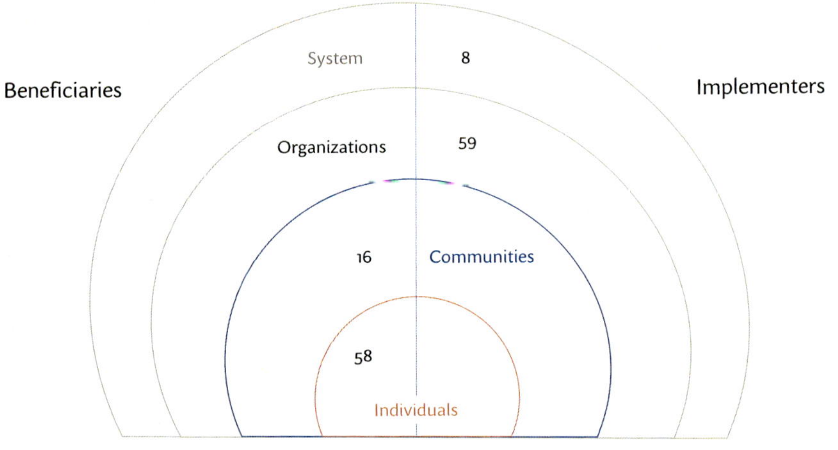

beneficiaries seen at the individual level (58 out of 74 citations; 78%). Implementers mapped to organization and system levels, with 59 of the 67 citations (88%) mapped to the organization level.

2.2.3 Evaluation of policy-related activities

Of the 46 policies identified, 28 policies (61%) stated plans for evaluation of some or all aspects of the policy, 15 (33%) did not describe any plans for evaluation and three were under development with no further details available. Of the 28 policies that stated plans for evaluation, 17 policies from 10 Member States had completed some or all of the planned evaluations, and the results were publically available.[3]

Activities had been evaluated using a range of methods, and several with more than one method (29,82–87). The commonest type of evaluation was the outcome evaluation, that is, confirmation that the target outcomes had been achieved.

3 Details of policy-related activities are available on request from euhen@who.int (Table 2. Policy-related activities).

One example is from an Austrian policy, Ensure the sustainability of communication and training in the care of people with disabilities (88), arising from the Austrian Health Literacy Platform (37). The activity resulted in the production of a so-called communication passport, containing all relevant information from health and social care professionals, carers, and the individual, demonstrating that the planned outcome had been achieved. Although useful, this does not provide any information on effectiveness; therefore, outcome evaluations are not considered further in this report. The other two types of evaluation were qualitative and quantitative methods; these were sometimes employed simultaneously. Both methods provide information on the effect of policies.

All evaluated activities were analysed using the Health Literacy Policy Model (Fig 4). Most mapped to the health services and education through the life-course vectors and within these to the individual, community (including family) and organization levels. Some activities also mapped to the lived environment and employment vectors. None of the evaluated activities mapped to the system level or to the media and digital/e-health vectors.

Fig. 4. Numbers of policy-related activities mapped to the four levels of the Health Literacy Policy Model

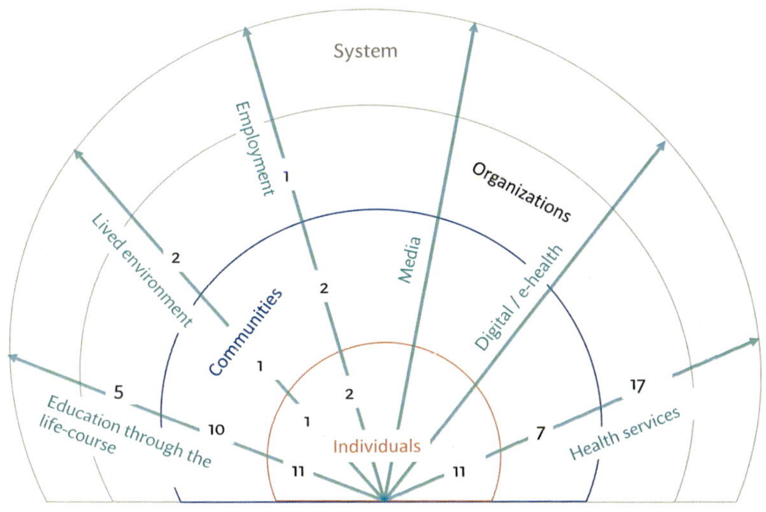

Policy-related activities with individual-level beneficiaries

Activities with evaluated results. Most evaluated activities at this level aimed to build health literacy in patients with chronic disease. All demonstrated tangible benefits for patients, with no negative outcomes reported. The Herzensbildung project (89) (linked to the Austrian national policy (37)) taught patients with heart disease about its prevention and management and supported the development of health literacy in heart disease, resulting in improved knowledge, improved confidence and reduced smoking in patients. In another activity focused on a specific health condition, patients at a local demonstrator site in England (90) (linked to English national policy (70)) who had poorly controlled diabetes were taught health literacy skills using a validated training programme developed in a previous policy, Skilled for Health (72). This resulted in increased patient knowledge, improved medication management and improved use of health care services. Some activities were not specific to a single health condition but instead focused on patients with any chronic illness. In Israel, an information prescription service to improve health literacy skills in patients resulted in high patient satisfaction and improved adherence to medication regimens (D Levin-Zamir, Clalit Services, Israel, personal communication, 13 March 2018; project arising from policy (53)). In Catalonia (Spain), the Prevention and Chronicity Attention programme (32) developed patient support groups using the Expert Patient Programme (91), resulting in improved quality of life, service utilization and self-care abilities for patients with chronic conditions (28). One evaluated policy activity aimed at individuals outside the health vector is the Finnish school education curriculum (42,92), which aimed to build health literacy in Finnish pupils throughout their school lives. This high-quality national assessment (described in Case study 1) enables education authorities to assess the effect of the teaching on pupils' skills.

Activities with evaluated results not yet available. Individual-level beneficiaries of these activities include patients, citizens and learners. Some activities are aimed to increase health literacy in patients and the general population (Germany (46), Italy (Umbria) (57) and Switzerland (68)) and others aim to improve digital/e-health literacy (Israel (53)). Some activities focus on education through the life-course; for example, in Puglia (Italy), health literacy is taught in schools, with the aim of reducing risky health behaviours (59). The German National decade for literacy and basic skills project aims to build health literacy in adults across society (48), and the Trentino (Italy) policy focuses on disease prevention through improving citizens' health literacy in relation to lifestyle, particularly in older people (56).

Case study 1. Quantitative evaluation of a Finnish national policy

A national evaluation of effects of the Finnish policy, Health education learning outcomes in basic education (92), on student learning from the national curriculum (42) assessed health literacy learning from year 1 (age 7 years) to year 9 (age 16 years), including health promotion, health protection, disease prevention and "health, communities and culture" (42). In Finland, all pupils are assessed in year 9 (age 16 years) and a national quantitative assessment is undertaken every 10 years (92). This evaluation has shown a satisfactory level of student development of health literacy across the curriculum.

Policy-related activities with community-level beneficiaries

Activities with evaluated results. Many of these activities focused on building health literacy in vulnerable groups. Examples are the MiMi project for migrants (Austria, Germany and Switzerland (37,50,69); described further in Case study 2) and the Swedish programme to build health literacy in migrants (33), of which a subproject focused on building sexual health literacy in migrant women (Case study 3) (27). In Israel, a local project within the national policy, Cultural appropriateness and accessibility (52), aimed to increase engagement with, and health access for, migrants. This project led to increased migrant participation in screening programmes, improved patient adherence to self-management programmes and better patient navigation of the health care system (D Levin-Zamir, Clalit Services, Israel, personal communication, 13 March 2018). An activity aimed at improving health literacy in a socially excluded group in Ireland, the Atelier Men's Roma Project (26), which arose from the Irish National Intercultural Health Strategy (30), led to increased health literacy, environmental safety (health and safety at work; fire safety in the home) and employment skills. Another activity focused on building health literacy skills in a disadvantaged community was the Stoke Speaks Out project (94), part of the English city-level policy Health Literacy Friendly Stoke (71). In this project, health literacy activities in early-years groups (children aged 0–5 years and their parents) in a socioeconomically deprived locality resulted in increased knowledge, language, skills and confidence in both children and parents in health-related areas such as going to the dentist or the doctor. In an Austrian activity aimed at building health literacy and health knowledge in overweight adolescents and their families, the Fit and Healthy project (95) (part of the national health literacy programme (37)), children/adolescents and their families were taught lifestyle skills, resulting in improved knowledge and action on exercise and diet. Another English policy, the Skilled for Health programme, aimed to build health literacy in disadvantaged communities by delivering training in multiple settings: socioeconomically deprived communities, workplaces with a high proportion of low-skilled workers, the army and prisons (72). The national evaluation demonstrated health literacy benefits through increased knowledge about health, illness, illness prevention and navigating health services. It also showed improvement in general literacy and numeracy skills and higher qualifications, leading to increased employability.

Activities with evaluated results not yet available. There is an early-years activity in Northern Ireland aimed at improving parenting skills, including in health literacy, and wider parental employment skills in socioeconomically deprived families with preschool children (73). Another policy-related activity in Italy (Umbria) aims to improve health through promoting cultural community activities (57).

Case study 2. The MiMi project – With Migrants for Migrants

The MiMi project was launched in 2003 as a pilot intervention in Germany (50), with financial support from the Federal Company of Health Insurance Funds (Betriebskrankenkasse Bundesverband). The intervention aims to address inequality in access to health care and health information among migrants by enhancing health literacy in the migrant population.

MiMi utilizes a peer mediator approach to ensure that health information is accessible and culturally appropriate. Migrants considered to be socially integrated, respected within their communities and well-educated receive approximately 50 hours of training as mediators, over evenings and weekends in topics including the health care system and key health care issues (e.g. sexual health, mental health, diet and nutrition, alcohol and tobacco consumption). The mediators promote health by conducting information-sharing events at places frequented by their peers and offer support and signposting to fellow migrants to enhance their personal health understanding and responsibility. Thus, the mediators "act as bridge builders between less well integrated migrants and the German health system" (50).

Evaluation of the project is ongoing; it includes questionnaires for mediators following training, qualitative interviews and a cost–benefit analysis. MiMi has received WHO approval, featuring as a case study on tackling poverty and social exclusion, and won the European Health Award in 2015 (93). The project

Case study 2. (contd)

has expanded to cover 64 locations in Germany and Austria (37) and has been utilized within the Swiss national programme on migration and health (69). MiMi is a key example of how Member States within the Region can learn from one another's initiatives and collaborate to improve both health and health care access for key population groups.

Case study 3. Qualitative study of health literacy in newly arrived refugee women in Sweden

In Sweden, newly arrived immigrants receive culturally sensitive health education (including on sexual health) in group settings (33). A qualitative study explored immigrant women's perspectives on the extent to which the health education had increased their sexual health literacy. The women interviewed reported improved knowledge about sexual health (including medical terminology), increased confidence in discussing sexual health issues with friends and family, increased awareness of their rights, and increased empowerment related to sexual health. Thus, health education had increased the women's functional, interactive and critical health literacy (27).

Policy-related activities with organization-level beneficiaries

Activities with evaluated results. Two policy-related activities that aimed to improve the health literacy competencies of those providing services for people with low health literacy were identified. In a national demonstrator site linked to the current English health literacy policy (70), a health literacy training programme for health, social care, fire and rescue, and community staff led to increased staff knowledge and confidence in supporting patients and clients (90). In a national demonstrator site in Scotland, staff training activities, such as use of the Teach-Back technique (96,97), led to improved staff confidence in meeting the needs of patients with low health literacy (98).

Activities with evaluated results not yet available. Several activities aim to improve the performance of organizations that provide services for people with low health literacy. In Valle D'Aosta (Italy), there is a focus on intercultural mediation services to improve health services for people from different cultural and ethnic groups (54). Some policies have activities to improve the clarity of health information and/or hospital signage (54,55,75) and the skills of health professionals (46,54,55,58). The German policy, National decade for literacy and basic skills (48), aims to build health literacy skills in teachers. Activities in the Trentino (Italy) policy involve the media and journalists (56).

Policy-related activities with system-level beneficiaries

Activities with evaluated results. None of the reported evaluated policy-related activities identified for this evidence synthesis explored system-level activities.

Activities with evaluated results not yet available. The German policy, National decade for literacy and basic skills, describes "establishing, developing and disseminating structures" (48), while the Irish Framework for improved health and wellbeing describes "incorporating health literacy into developing health and education policy" (51). Evaluation of these activities is anticipated to produce valuable information on the effectiveness of these system-level activities.

Health literacy portals

Activities resulting in publically accessible portals containing health literacy information and tools were found arising from policies in Austria (37), Germany (31,48), the Russian Federation (63) and the United Kingdom (70,72,75).

2.2.4 Factors influencing policy effectiveness

Information on the factors (i.e. facilitators and barriers) influencing the successful implementation of health literacy policy was obtained from the peer-reviewed literature (34–36), which explored the views of policy-makers who had developed and implemented policies, including health literacy policies, as part of the WHO Health Cities Network (99).

Facilitators. In an analysis of 112 case studies, Green et al. showed that over 90% referred to five prerequisites (based on Tsouros (100)): intersectoral working, supportive institutional structures and processes, political leadership, community participation and networking (35). The importance of intersectoral working was shown in Stavropol (Russian Federation), where the programme for preventing noncommunicable diseases drew on expertise from the State Medical University and involved the municipal departments of health care, education and social protection (35). The importance of political leadership was highlighted by Morrison et al.: a participant from Lisbon commented that "tackling inequalities in health should be a priority in the Lisbon Metropolitan

Area and is not, directly, (this is) a hotly debated topic" (34). Several authors commented on the benefits of engaging and working with communities. For example, Green et al. described a policy from Preston (United Kingdom) in which community control over certain streets made residents more aware of the health benefits of walking and socializing (35).

Barriers. The barriers to successful policies included cultural barriers. For example, Morrison et al. reported that informants from Stockholm and Lisbon considered the obstacles addressing health inequalities to be essentially related to embedded cultural beliefs, which made adopting healthier lifestyles difficult (34). Budget restrictions were also important: the same study reported that "a very important one is the financial issue. Every year we have less money and the crisis only makes it worse" (34). Another reported barrier was the difficulty obtaining high-quality evidence: Bull et al. found that the presence and use of such evidence varied considerably (36).

3. DISCUSSION

3.1 Strengths and limitations

This review analysed the identified health literacy policy policies using a clear framework. Although languages in the core team were restricted to Dutch, English and German, the review team collaborated with speakers of several additional European languages (Catalan, Finnish, French, Greek, Hebrew, Italian, Portuguese, Russian and Spanish) through extensive networks. Preliminary findings were presented to the inaugural meeting of the WHO European Health Information Initiative Action Network on Measuring Health Literacy (22–23 February 2018) (101), attended by representatives from 19 Member States, who had the opportunity to alert the lead author to gaps and errors in the report and advise on its usefulness for future decisions and actions. In addition, expert enquiries were made to various stakeholders including enquiries in Russian to the countries in the Commonwealth of Independent States (Armenia, Azerbaijan, Belarus, Kazakhstan, Kyrgyzstan, Republic of Moldova, Tajikistan and Uzbekistan); however, no response was received from any of these countries.

Some of the regional and national policy briefs, statements and guidelines that did not meet the precise definition of health policy were not included in the evidence synthesis; however, these are cited as background material contributing to the current political and organizational environment within which policies can be developed and delivered.

Many important health literacy activities not linked with policy, such as primary research and community activities, were not included in this evidence synthesis. Of the 15 300 peer-reviewed publications identified in the literature search, only four could be directly linked to one or more policies, with another three exploring policy-related barriers and facilitators; this compares with 2447 publications cited on PubMed in the years 2008 to 2017 with the term **health literacy** in the title, of which a significant proportion of these remaining publications could be expected to describe health literacy activities from the WHO European Region. An evidence synthesis of these non-policy-related activities would form a useful future Health Evidence Network synthesis report.

3.2 Policy considerations

Increasing recognition of the importance of health literacy in delivering health and health equity (11) and its importance in delivering the health strategy of the WHO European Region, Health 2020 (8), requires a more systematic approach to the development of health literacy policy and to evaluation of their effectiveness in Member States. This report highlights good practice and emerging evidence of effectiveness of health literacy policies for patients, citizens and communities, but also shows that policies could benefit from a more holistic approach.

The following policy considerations are proposed to Member States:

- consider the existing policies and related activities gathered in review to develop or enhance health literacy policies and related activities to benefit citizens, patients and communities;
- broaden the range of areas of activity required for holistic health literacy policies to include the lived environment, the workplace, the media and digital/e-health, at all societal levels – individual, community, organization and system (legislative);
- strengthen the evidence base for health literacy at all societal levels to ensure that policies address needs specific to the national or local context;
- incorporate robust qualitative and quantitative evaluations into health literacy policies and interventions – quantitative methods could include pre- and post-activity health literacy evaluations of evidence of health, social and economic effects at all levels; and
- incorporate facilitators of successful implementation, such as intersectoral working, political leadership and strategies to overcome cultural barriers, into health literacy policy.

Better engagement between policy-makers and the academic community would be helpful in gathering robust data to inform policy and to evaluate the effectiveness of policy-related activities. The newly instituted European Health Information Initiative's Action Network on Measuring Population and Organizational Health Literacy (101), which brings together policy-makers and academic researchers, provides an excellent opportunity to realize this.

4. CONCLUSIONS

Health literacy has been recognized as a means to promote health, reduce the risk of illness and premature death, and promote cost-effective, person-centred, equitable health care. Central to health literacy is the development of skills through the life-course, including preschool activities, formal instruction in schools and adult learning. Other key aspects are the health service, the lived environment, employment, the media and digital health. Health literacy has been recognized as the key to developing policies that are effective in improving health, improving the effectiveness of health systems and promoting equity.

This report identified a wide range of health literacy policies and policy-related activities in the WHO European Region. However, it also identified gaps in geography; health literacy metrics and evidence of health, social and economic effects of policies; the breadth of societal areas addressed in the policies; and intersectoral activities. The policy considerations outlined, if adopted, would promote the development of holistic health literacy policies in Member States and the development, implementation and rigorous evaluation of policy-related activities to demonstrate the benefits of health literacy policies to citizens and society.

REFERENCES

1. World Health Organization [website]. Copenhagen: WHO Regional Office for Europe; 2017 (http://www.euro.who.int/en/about-us/organization, accessed 31 December 2017).
2. Development Assistance Committee. DAC list of ODA recipients: effective for reporting on 2014, 2015 and 2016 flows. Paris: Organization for Economic Co-operation and Development; 2017 (http://www.oecd.org/dac/stats/documentupload/DAC_List_ODA_Recipients2014to2017_flows_En.pdf, accessed 9 November 2017).
3. Sørensen K, Van den Broucke S, Fullam J, Doyle G, Pelikan J, Slonska Z et al. Health literacy and public health: a systematic review and integration of definitions and models. BMC Public Health. 2012;12:80.
4. Political declaration of the High-level Meeting of the General Assembly Sørensen K, Pelikan JM, Röthlin F, Ganahl K, Slonska Z, Doyle G et al. Health literacy in Europe: comparative results of the European health literacy survey (HLS-EU). Eur J Public Health. 2015;25(6):1053–8.
5. Heijmans M, Uiters E, Rose T, Hofstede J, Devillé W, van der Heide I et al. Study on sound evidence for a better understanding of health literacy in the European Union (HEALIT4EU): final report. Luxembourg: Publications Office of the European Union; 2015.
6. Berkman ND, Sheridan SL, Donahue KE, Halpern DJ, Viera A, Crotty K et al. Health literacy interventions and outcomes: an updated systematic review. Rockville (MD): Agency for Health Care Research and Quality (US); 2011.
7. Robertson R, Wenzel L, Thompson J, Charles A. Understanding NHS financial pressures: how are they affecting patient care? London: King's Fund; 2017 (https://www.kingsfund.org.uk/sites/default/files/field/field_publication_file/Understanding NHS financial pressures - full report.pdf, accessed 10 March 2018).
8. Health 2020: a European policy framework and strategy for the 21st century. Copenhagen: WHO Regional Office for Europe; 2013 (http://www.euro.who.int/en/publications/policy-documents/health-2020.-a-european-policy-framework-and-strategy-for-the-21st-century-2013, accessed 10 March 2018).
9. Eichler K, Wieser S, Brugger U. The costs of limited health literacy: a systematic review. Int J Public Health. 2009;54(5):313–24.

10. Vandenbosch J, Van den Broucke S, Vancorenland S, Avalosse H, Verniest R, Callens M. Health literacy and the use of healthcare services in Belgium. J Epidemiol Community Health. 2016;70(10):1032–8.

11. The Shanghai Declaration on promoting health in the 2030 Agenda for Sustainable Development. Geneva: World Health Organization; 2016 (9th Global Conference on Health Promotion).

12. Quaglio G, Sørensen K, Rübig P, Bertinato L, Brand H, Karapiperis T et al. Accelerating the health literacy agenda in Europe. Health Promot Int. 2017;32(6):1074–80.

13. McDaid D. Investing in health literacy. Copenhagen: WHO Regional Office for Europe; 2016.

14. Sustainable health systems for inclusive growth in Europe. Geneva: World Health Organization; 2018 (http://www.euro.who.int/en/health-topics/Health-systems/pages/news/news/2013/11/sustainable-health-systems-for-inclusive-growth-in-europe, accessed 5 March 2018).

15. The Riga roadmap. Investing in health and wellbeing for all. Riga: Latvian Presidency of the Council of the European Union; 2015 (Universal Health Care Conference; http://rigahealthconference2015.eu/wp-content/uploads/2015/08/Riga-Roadmap-download-FINAL.pdf, accessed 5 March 2018).

16. The Minsk Declaration. The life-course approach in the context of Health 2020. Copenhagen: WHO Regional Office for Europe; 2015 (http://www.euro.who.int/__data/assets/pdf_file/0009/289962/The-Minsk-Declaration-EN-rev1.pdf?ua=1, accessed 14 March 2018).

17. Paris Declaration. Partnerships for the health and well-being of our young and future generations. Copenhagen: WHO Regional Office for Europe; 2016 (http://www.euro.who.int/__data/assets/pdf_file/0019/325180/Paris_Declaration_ENG.pdf?ua=1, accessed 14 March 2018).

18. 2017 Healthy Cities Pécs Declaration. Copenhagen: WHO Regional Office for Europe; 2017 (http://www.euro.who.int/__data/assets/pdf_file/0005/334643/Pecs-Declaration.pdf, accessed 14 March 2018).

19. Health literacy: the solid facts. Copenhagen: WHO Regional Office for Europe; 2013.

20. Gesundheitskompetenz fördern – Ansätze und Impulse. Ein Action Guide der Allianz Gesundheitskompetenz. Bern: Allianz Gesundheitskompetenz; 2016 (http://www.allianz-gesundheitskompetenz.ch/logicio/client/allianz/file/Literatur/Brosch_A4_Gesundheitskompetenz_dt_web.pdf, accessed 5 March 2018).

21. Gesundheitskompetenz in der Schweiz – Stand und Perspektiven. Bern: Allianz Gesundheitskompetenz; 2015 (http://www.allianz-gesundheitskompetenz.ch/logicio/client/allianz/file/Literatur/Gesundheitskompetenz__Sammelband.pdf, accessed 10 March 2018).

22. Kickbusch I, Wait S, Magg D. Navigating health. The role of health literacy. London: Alliance for Health and the Future; 2005.

23. Pleasant A. Appendix A. Health literacy around the world: part 1. Health literacy efforts outside of the United States. In: Health literacy: improving health, health systems, and health policy around the world: workshop summary. Washington (DC): Institute of Medicine; 2013.

24. Health education: theoretical concepts, effective strategies and core competencies; a foundation document to guide capacity development of health educators. Cairo: WHO Regional Office for the Eastern Mediterranean; 2012.

25. Health policy. Geneva: World Health Organization; 2018 (http://www.who.int/topics/health_policy/en/, accessed 15 January 2018).

26. Evaluation of the Atelier Roma Men's Training, Diversion and Health Literacy Programme. Dublin: Health Service Executive; 2016 (http://www.hse.ie/eng/about/Who/primarycare/socialinclusion/intercultural-health/Atelier-Report.pdf, accessed 10 January 2018).

27. Svensson P, Carlzen K, Agardh A. Exposure to culturally sensitive sexual health information and impact on health literacy: a qualitative study among newly arrived refugee women in Sweden. Cult Health Sex. 2016;19(7):752–66.

28. Bujan PA, González Mestre A, Blay Pueyo C, Ledesma Castelltort A, Contel Segura JC, Constante Beitia C. Expert Patient Programme Catalonia: a person-centered community perspective. Int J Integr Care. 2015;15(Annu Conf Suppl): URN:NBN:NL:UI:10-1-117086.

29. Gromnica-Ihle E, Faubel U, Cattelaens K. [How does the German Association against Rheumatism and Arthritis convey health literacy?] Z Rheumatol. 2014;73(8):721–8 (in German).

30. National intercultural health strategy 2007–2012. Dublin: Health Service Executive; 2008 (https://www.hse.ie/eng/services/publications/socialinclusion/national-intercultural-health-strategy-2007---2012.pdf, accessed 6 January 2018).

31. Leitbild der Deutschen Rheuma-Liga. Bonn: Deutsche Rheuma-Liga Bundesverband e.V.; 2014 (https://www.rheuma-liga.de/fileadmin/user_upload/Dokumente/Verband/Leitbild/DRL_Leitbild_final.pdf, accessed 6 March 2018).

32. Programa de prevenció i`atenció a la cronicitat [Prevention and chronicity attention programme]. Barcelona: Departament de Salut, Generalitat de Catalunya; 2012 (in Catalonian; http://salutweb.gencat.cat/web/.content/home/ambits_tematics/linies_dactuacio/model_assistencial/atencio_al_malalt_cronic/documents/arxius/562conceptual.pdf, accessed 10 March 2018).

33. Lag om etableringsinsatser för nyanlända invandrare [Law on introduction of activities for newly arrived immigrants]. Stockholm: Swedish Parliament; 2010 (in Swedish; http://www.riksdagen.se/sv/dokument-lagar/dokument/svensk-forfattningssamling/lag-2010197-om-etableringsinsatserfor-vissa_sfs-2010-197, accessed 5 March 2017).

34. Morrison J, Pons-Vigués M, Bécares L, Burström B, Gandarillas A, Domínguez-Berjón F et al. Health inequalities in European cities: perceptions and beliefs among local policymakers. BMJ Open. 2014;4(5):e004454.

35. Green G, Jackisch J, Zamaro G. Healthy cities as catalysts for caring and supportive environments. Health Promot Int. 2015;30(suppl 1):99–107.

36. Bull F, Milton K, Kahlmeier S, Arlotti A, Juričan AB, Belander O et al. Turning the tide: national policy approaches to increasing physical activity in seven European countries. Br J Sports Med. 2015;49(11):749–56.

37. Gesundheitsziele Österreich. In: Austrian health literacy platform [website]. Vienna: Federal Ministry of Health and Women's Affairs; 2016 (https://oepgk.at/, accessed 10 March 2018).

38. Session de 2016–2017. Brussels: Sénat de Belgique; 2017 (https://www.senate.be/www/?MIval=/index_senate&MENUID=12410&LANG=fr, accessed 10 May 2018).

39. Strateški plan razvoja javnog zdravstva 2013–2015 [Strategic development plan for public health 2013–2015]. Zagreb: Ministry of Health of the Republic of Croatia; 2013 (in Croatian; http://hzzzsr.hr/wp-content/uploads/2017/03/Strateski-plan-javnog-zdravstva-2013-2015.pdf, accessed 10 March 2018).

40. Plan za zdravlje i socijalno blagostanje Primorsko-Goranske Zupanye za Radzdoblje 2015–2018 [Plan for health and social well-being of Primorje-Gorski County 2015–2018]. Rijeka: Primorje-Gorski County Assembly; 2015 (in Croatian; http://www2.pgz.hr/doc/dokumenti/03-plan-zdravlje.pdf, accessed 10 March 2018).

41. Health 2020: national strategy for health protection and promotion and disease prevention (Czech Republic). Prague: Ministry of Health of the Czech Republic; 2014.

42. Perusopetuksen opetussuunnitelman perusteet; terveystieto [National core curriculum for basic education; health education]. Helsinki: Education FNAf; 2014 (in Finnish).
43. La stratégie nationale de santé 2018–2022. Paris: Ministère des Solidarités et de la Santé. 2017 (http://solidarites-sante.gouv.fr/systeme-de-sante-et-medico-social/strategie-nationale-de-sante/article/la-strategie-nationale-de-sante-2018-2022, accessed 10 March 2018).
44. Plan d'actions de prevention et de lutte contre l'illettrisme 2011–2015. Sant Denis (Reunion, France): Caref-Orer Reunion; 2011 (http://www.cariforef-reunion.net/index.php?option=com_content&view=article&id=752:plan-d-actions-de-prevention-et-de-lutte-contre-l-illettrisme-a-la-reunion-agir-pour-lire-lire-pour-agir-2011-2015&catid=177&Itemid=1163, accessed 10 March 2018).
45. Pays de la Loire programme régional d'accès à la prévention et aux soins (PRAPS) 2012–2016. Nantes: Agence Regionale de Picardie et Projet Regionale de Sante de Picardie; 2012 (http://www.crsa-pays-de-la-loire.ars.sante.fr/fileadmin/PAYS-LOIRE/F_concertation_regionale/prs/prs-mars-2012/pdf/5-1-Programme-Regional-d_Acces-a-la-Prevention-et-aux-Soins-PRAPS.pdf, accessed 10 March 2018).
46. Nationaler Aktionsplan Gesundheitskompetenz. Berlin: Hertie School of Governance and Universität Bielefeld; 2018 (http://www.nap-gesundheitskompetenz.de/, accessed 10 March 2018).
47. Übersicht über aktuelle Maßnahmen der Partner der Allianz für Gesundheitskompetenz. Berlin: Bundesministerium für Gesundheit; 2017 (https://www.bundesgesundheitsministerium.de/fileadmin/Dateien/3_Downloads/G/Gesundheit/Allianz_Gesundheitskompetenz_Massnahmen.pdf, accessed 10 December 2017).
48. Grundsatzpapier zur Nationalen Dekade für Alphabetisierung und Grundbildung 2016–2026. Berlin: Bundesministerium für Bildung und Forschung; 2018 (https://www.alphadekade.de/files/01_Grundsatzpapier zur Nationalen Dekade Alphabetisierung und Grundbildung_final.pdf, accessed 6 March 2018).
49. Gesundheitliche Kompetenz erhöhen, Patient(inn)ensouveränität stärken (2003; Aktualisierung 2011). Berlin: Gesunddheitsziele.de; 2011 (http://gesundheitsziele.de/cgi-bin/render.cgi?__cms_page=nationale_gz, accessed 6 March 2018).
50. Was ist MiMi? [website]. Hanover: Ethno Medizinisches Zentrum e.V.; 2017 (https://www.mimi-bestellportal.de/was-ist-mimi/, accessed 10 March 2018).

51. Healthy Ireland. A framework for improved health and wellbeing 2013–2025. Dublin: Department of Health; 2013 (http://health.gov.ie/wp-content/uploads/2014/03/HealthyIrelandBrochureWA2.pdf, accessed 10 March 2018).
52. Cultural appropriateness and accessibility of the healthcare system. Jerusalem: Ministry of Health; 2011 (in Hebrew).
53. Health literacy workplan. Health Literacy Section, Department of Health Education and Promotion 2017–2018. Tel Aviv 2017: Clalit Health Services.
54. Sviluppo di un Programma di Health Literacy: Leggere, capire e comunicare le informazioni per la salute [Development of a programme of health literacy: read, understand and communicate about health]. Aosta: Valle D'Aosta Local Health Authority; 2013 (in Italian).
55. Capirsi fa bene alla salute [Understanding each other is good for health]. In: Piano sociale e sanitario dell'Emilia-Romagna 2017–2019 [Social and health plan of Emilia-Romagna 2017–2019]. Bologna: Information and Communication Agency of the Regional Council of Emilia-Romagna; 2017 (in Italian; http://salute.regione.emilia-romagna.it/ssr/piano-sociale-e-sanitario/piano-sociale-e-sanitario-la-programmazione, accessed 15 December 2017).
56. Piano per la salute del Trentino 2015–2020 [Plan for the health of Trentino 2015–2025]. Trento: Department of Health and Social Solidarity; 2015 (in Italian; https://partecipa.tn.it/uploads/pianosalute/piano-per-la-salute-del-trentino-2015-2025.pdf, accessed 15 December 2017).
57. Piano regional di prevenzione Umbria 2014–2018 [Regional prevention plan for Umbria 2014–2018]. Perugia: Il Consiglio Regionale dell'Umbria; 2014 (in Italian; http://www.regione.umbria.it/documents/18/3195498/Allegato+1+PRP+2014+2018+Parte+2_prova+web_pagine.pdf/4d07762a-25c6-4c1c-a6e7-51af7bcfeda3, accessed 15 December 2017).
58. Piano sanitario e sociale integrato regionale (Tuscano) 2012–2015 [Health and social care integrated plan (Tuscany) 2012–2015]. Florence: Il Consiglio Regionale della Toscana; 2012 (in Italian).
59. Piano strategico regionale per la promozione all salute nella scuole 2017–2018 [Regional strategic plan for health promotion in schools 2017–2018]. Bari: Regione Puglia Assessorato alla Salute; 2017 (in Italian; https://www.sanita.puglia.it/documents/20182/26611972/Catalogo+Salute+Scuola+2017-18/f1b3f2bb-da30-4795-88e1-5b76eaf2e9f8, accessed 15 December 2017).

60. Programa nacional de educação para a saúde, literacia e autocuidados [National programme for education and health literacy and self-care]. Lisbon: Directorate-General for Health; 2016 (Contract no. 49; in Portuguese; https://www.dgs.pt/em-destaque/programa-nacional-de-educacao-para-a-saude-literacia-e-autocuidados.aspx, accessed 10 March 2018).

61. Elaborarea materialelor de informare şi educare pentru promovarea sănătăţii şi educaţie pentru sănătate [Elaboration of information and education materials to promote health and health education]. Bucharest: Şcoala Naţională de Sănătate Publică şi Management Sanitar; 2006 (in Romanian).

62. Planul Multianual Integrat de Promovare a Sănătăţii şi Educaţie pentru Sănătate [Multiannual integrated plan for health promotion and education for health]. Bucharest: Ministry of Health; 2016 (in Romanian; http://old.ms.ro/upload/plan-integrat-tipar_mic-ultima-versiune.pdf, accessed 10 March 2018).

63. Проект Стратегии формирования здорового образа жизни населения, профилактики и контроля неинфекционных заболеваний на период до 2025 года [Draft strategy on healthy lifestyle promotion, prevention and control of non-communicable diseases for the period until 2025]. Moscow: Department of Health 2018 (in Russian).

64. Piano sanitario e sociosanitario della Repubblica di San Marino 2015–2017 [Health and sanitary plan of the Republic of San Marino 2015–2017]. San Marino: State Secretariat for Health and Social Security, Family, Security and Economic Planning; 2015 (in Italian).

65. Osebna odgovornost za zdravje in dolžnosti posameznikov glede zdravja in zdravstva [Personal responsibility for the health and duties of individuals with regard to health and health]. Ljubljana: Institute for Health Care of Slovenia; 2017 (in Slovene; http://www.zzzs.si/novosti/5A5960D1EB7845AEC12581AF0041568A?open&l=p, accessed 20 November 2018).

66. Pla de salut 2016–2020 [Health plan of Catalonia 2016/2020]. Barcelona: Government of Catalonia; 2017 (in Catalonian; http://salutweb.gencat.cat/ca/el_departament/Pla_salut/pla-de-salut-2016–2020/, accessed 10 March 2018).

67. IV Plan de salud de la Comunidad Valenciana (2016/2020) [IV Health plan of the region of Valencia (2016–2020)]. Valencia: Government of Valencia; 2016 (in Spanish; http://www.san.gva.es/documents/157385/6431837/IV_PLAN+DE+SALUD_CV_2016_Castellano_web.pdf, accessed 10 March 2018).

68. Nationale Strategie zur Prävention nichtübertragbarer Krankheiten. Bern: Federal Office of Public Health; 2018 (https://www.bag.admin.ch/bag/de/home/themen/strategien-politik/nationale-gesundheitsstrategien/strategie-nicht-uebertragbare-krankheiten.html, accessed 5 March 2018).

69. National programme on migration and health: 2008–2013 results and priorities for 2014–2017. Bern: Federal Office of Public Health; 2013.

70. Enabling people to make informed health decisions. Health literacy [website]. Leeds: NHS England; 2018 (https://www.england.nhs.uk/ourwork/patient-participation/health-decisions/, accessed 9 March 2018).

71. "Health literacy friendly" Stoke-on-Trent. Stoke-on-Trent: Stoke-on-Trent City Council; 2017.

72. Evaluation of the second phase of the Skilled for Health programme. London: The Tavistock Institute and Shared Intelligence; 2009.

73. Making life better. A whole system strategic framework for public health 2013–2023. Belfast: Department of Health, Social Services and Public Safety; 2014 (https://www.health-ni.gov.uk/sites/default/files/publications/dhssps/making-life-better-strategic-framework-2013-2023_0.pdf, accessed 10 March 2018).

74. Belfast Healthy Cities: health literacy. Belfast: Belfast City Council; 2015 (https://www.belfasthealthycities.com/what-health-literacy, accessed 31 December 2017).

75. Making it easy: a health literacy plan for Scotland. Edinburgh: NHS Scotland; 2014 (http://www.gov.scot/Resource/0045/00451263.pdf, accessed 15 November 2017).

76. Making it easier: a health literacy action plan 2017–2025. Edinburgh: NHS Scotland; 2017 (https://beta.gov.scot/publications/making-easier-health-literacy-action-plan-scotland-2017-2025/documents/00528139.pdf?inline=true, accessed 6 January 2018).

77. Fairer health outcomes for all. Reducing inequities in health strategic action plan. Cardiff: Welsh Assembly Government; 2011 (http://www.wales.nhs.uk/sitesplus/documents/866/5.1 Appendix Fairer Outcomes for All-Welsh Assembly Government Document.pdf, accessed 15 November 2017).

78. The Abertawe Bro Morgannwg University Health Board health literacy policy. Swansea: Abertawe Bro Morgannwg University Health Board; 2017.

79. Benoit F. Public policy models and their usefulness in public health: the Stages Model. Montréal (Québec): National Collaborating Centre for Healthy Public Policy; 2013 (http://www.ncchpp.ca/docs/ModeleEtapesPolPubliques_EN.pdf, accessed 19 March 2018).

80. Cheung KK, Mirzaei M, Leeder S. Health policy analysis: a tool to evaluate in policy documents the alignment between policy statements and intended outcomes. Aust Health Rev. 2010;34(4):405–13.

81. Norman CD, Skinner HA. eHealth literacy: essential skills for consumer health in a networked world. J Med Internet Res. 2006;8(2):e9.

82. The health literacy place [website]. Edinburgh: NHS Scotland; 2017 (http://www.healthliteracyplace.org.uk/learning-and-development/national-training-courses/nhs-education-for-scotland/, accessed 10 March 2018).

83. Positive health – cooperate, participate, be active! In: Austrian health literacy platform [website]. Vienna: Federal Ministry of Health and Women's Affairs; 2016 (https://oepgk.at/massnahmen/positive-health/, accessed 10 March 2018).

84. Gesundheit kommt nachhause: Interkulturelle Gesundheitsförderung in aufsuchender Bildungsarbeit für Migrantinnen und ihre Kinder im Vor- und Pflichtschulalter. Vienna: Beratungsgruppe.at; 2011 (http://www.gekona.at/index.php?SID=327, accessed 17 December 2017).

85. A health literacy walk-through. Addressing health literacy issues in accessing and engaging with health services: navigation of the hospital environment. In: The health literacy place [website]. Edinburgh: NHS Scotland; 2016 (http://www.healthliteracyplace.org.uk/blog/2016/news/health-literacy-demonstrator-site-headline-report-one/, accessed 31 December 2017).

86. Meaningful communication before medical procedures. In: The health literacy place [website]. Edinburgh: NHS Scotland; 2016 (http://www.healthliteracyplace.org.uk/blog/2017/news/health-literacy-demonstrator-site-headline-report-three/, accessed 10 March 2018).

87. Making it easy – progress against actions. Edinburgh: NHS Scotland; 2017 (http://www.gov.scot/Publications/2017/07/7806/downloads, accessed 23 April 2018).

88. Sicherung der Nachhaltigkeit von Kommunikations- und Fortbildungsmaßnahmen in der Gesundheitsversorgung von Menschen mit Behinderungen. In: Austrian health literacy platform [website]. Vienna: Federal Ministry of Health and Women's Affairs; 2018 (https://oepgk.at/massnahmen/geko-wien/, accessed 2018 10 March).

89. Herzensbildung. In: Austrian health literacy platform [website]. Vienna: Federal Ministry of Health and Women's Affairs; 2016 (https://oepgk.at/massnahmen/herzensbildung/, accessed 10 March 2018).

90. Making the case for health literacy: East Midlands national demonstrator site 2016–17. Strategic report. Leeds: Health Education England; 2017 (https://www.hee.nhs.uk/our-work/health-literacy, accessed 10 May 2018).

91. Lorig KR, Sobel DS, Ritter PL, Laurent D, Hobbs M. Effect of a self-management program on patients with chronic disease. Eff Clin Pract. 2001;4(6):256–62.
92. Terveystiedon oppimistulokset perusopetuksen päättövaiheessa [Health education learning outcomes in basic education]. Helsinki: Board of Education; 2013 (in Finnish).
93. Salman R, Weyers S. Germany. MiMi project – with migrants for migrants. Poverty and social exclusion in the WHO European Region: health systems respond. Copenhagen: WHO Regional Office for Europe; 2010:52–63.
94. Bailey V, Cheadle D. School readiness – Stoke speaks out. Stoke-on-Trent: Stoke-on Trent City Council; 2016 (http://webapps.stoke.gov.uk/uploadedfiles/Health-literacy-event-June-2016-reduced-file.pdf, accessed 10 March 2018).
95. Fit und Gsund. In: Austrian health literacy platform [website]. Vienna: Federal Ministry of Health and Women's Affairs; 2017 (https://oepgk.at/massnahmen/fit-und-gsund/, accessed 10 March 2018).
96. Tool 5. The Teach-Back method. Chapel Hill (NC): North Carolina Program on Health Literacy; 2015 (http://www.nchealthliteracy.org/toolkit/tool5.pdf, accessed 10 March 2018).
97. Developing checklists to remind and confirm the use of Teach-Back. In: The health literacy place [website]. Edinburgh: NHS Scotland; 2017 (http://www.healthliteracyplace.org.uk/blog/2017/news/health-literacy-demonstrator-site-headline-report-five/, accessed 10 March 2018).
98. Experiences of healthcare staff using Teach-Back in practice. In: The health literacy place [website]. Edinburgh: NHS Scotland; 2017 (http://www.healthliteracyplace.org.uk/blog/2017/professional-blogs/health-literacy-demonstrator-site-headline-report-six/, accessed 10 March 2018).
99. Healthy cities. Copenhagen: WHO Regional Office for Europe; 2018 (http://www.euro.who.int/en/health-topics/environment-and-health/urban-health/activities/healthy-cities, accessed 14 March 2018).
100. Tsouros A. City leadership for health and well-being: back to the future. J Urban Health. 2013;90(suppl 1):4–13.
101. European Health Information Initiative action network on measuring health literacy (http://www.uzg.cz/doc/Minutes-M-POHL.pdf, accessed 17 April 2018).

ANNEX 1. SEARCH AND ANALYSIS STRATEGY

Databases, websites and other sources

Searches and other evidence-gathering activities were conducted between 9 October 2017 and 20 January 2018.

The following databases were searched for academic peer-reviewed literature in Dutch, English and German using defined search terms: CINAHL (Cumulative Index to Nursing and Allied Health Literature), EMBASE, MEDLINE, PsycINFO and Web of Science. The strategy was kept broad to ensure all relevant documents were identified.

An Internet search of grey literature in English, Catalan, Dutch, French, German, Italian, Russian and Spanish was conducted in Google using a pre-defined search strategy developed by the research team and based on a previous successful search strategy used in the HEALIT4EU report (1).

The searches were supplemented by engagement with experts in known networks (the United Kingdom Health Literacy Collaborative (2), Health Literacy UK (3), the Health Literacy Global Working Group of the International Union for Health Promotion and Education (4), the Dutch Health Literacy Alliance (5), the Nordic Health Literacy Network (6) and the European Network of Health Promoting Schools (7)) and collaboration with speakers of several additional European languages (Finnish, Greek, Hebrew, Portuguese and Spanish) through extensive networks to identify additional documents. A snowball technique was used in which recipients were asked to forward the enquiry email to relevant contacts. Emails in Russian requesting information on policies were sent from the Russian Federation Ministry of Health to the ministries of health in the countries of the Commonwealth of Independent States (Armenia, Azerbaijan, Belarus, Kazakhstan, Kyrgyzstan, Republic of Moldova, Tajikistan and Uzbekistan). A draft of the report was presented to the inaugural meeting of the European Health Information Network Action Network on Measuring Health Literacy, to enable identification of missing policies and any errors in reporting.

Health literacy activities in the EU described in the recent HEALI4EU report (1) were independently reviewed (GR and JR) and seven meeting the synthesis review criteria were identified.

All searches included the term **health literacy** in English and translated into Dutch, French, German and Italian. All expert enquiry responses were in English.

Study selection

The results of all database searches were downloaded and combined into a single database. After duplicate removal, the titles and abstracts were screened for eligibility using the following inclusion and exclusion criteria and then reviewed by four researchers (GR, SS, EK and JR) to identify papers for final inclusion. Any areas of disagreement were resolved by discussion.

Inclusion criteria:

- could be classified as a health literacy policy as defined in this report (i.e. decisions, plans and actions undertaken to achieve specific health literacy goals within a society) or reported an activity arising from an identified policy;
- included the term **health literacy** (or the equivalent in the national language); and
- came from one of the 53 countries in the WHO European Region.

Exclusion criteria:

- not classified as policy, or activities arising from policy, according to the criteria used in this evidence synthesis;
- did not include the term **health literacy** (or the equivalent in the national language); or
- came from a country outside the Region.

Health literacy policies were identified from 19 Member States: Austria, Belgium, Croatia, Czechia, Finland, France, Germany, Ireland, Israel, Italy, Portugal, Romania, the Russian Federation, San Marino, Slovenia, Spain, Sweden, Switzerland and the United Kingdom.

Data extraction

The identified policies and papers were analysed using a synthesis framework developed during this review. Materials in Dutch, English or German were analysed by the authors; documents in other languages were analysed by native speakers recruited from the authors' academic departments and through the expert enquiry.

A quality check was undertaken by three authors (SR, AO'D and AT) on 5% of the titles identified in the initial search.

The synthesis framework was developed to identify:

- the country within which policy was based;
- the current status of the policy (active/completed/under development);
- the organizational level of the policy, classified as regional (i.e. Region level), national (i.e. Member State level or at the level of devolved strategy and funding for health) or local (i.e. at the level of a locality, a city or an organization);
- actors in the policy;
- the measures (i.e. actions) to be undertaken;
- the setting; and
- whether the policy resulted in a public health portal, through which health literacy information or tools could be publically accessed.

A draft version of the report was presented to the inaugural meeting of the WHO European Health Information Initiative Action Network on Measuring Health Literacy (22–23 February 2018) (8), where representatives from 19 Member States had the opportunity to highlight gaps and errors in the report and advise on its usefulness for future decisions and actions.

Search terms

The following terms were used for the PubMed search strategy. Other search strategies used these terms with minor modifications.

(((health adj literacy).mp. OR (Health Education/ OR Health Knowledge, Attitudes, Practice/ OR Health Literacy/) OR (Health literacy.mp. OR exp Health Literacy/) OR (health adj knowledge).mp. OR (medical adj data adj interpretation).mp. OR (health adj competence).mp. OR (gezondheidsvaardigheden OR gesundheitskompetenz).mp. OR (literacy OR literate OR reading OR writing OR numeracy).mp. OR (literacy.mp. OR Literacy/ OR Information Literacy/) OR ((reading adj level) OR (reading adj ability) OR (reading adj skills)).mp. OR ((writing adj ability) OR (writing adj level) OR (writing adj skills)).mp. OR analphabetism.mp.) AND ((Policy.mp. OR Health Policy/ OR Policy/ OR Public Policy/) OR (health adj care adj policy).mp. OR (programme OR programmes OR program OR programs).mp. OR (Health Planning/ OR health care planning.mp. OR Health Services Accessibility/) OR (health adj care adj planning).mp. OR (regulation OR (Public adj Health) OR strategy OR (Action adj plan) OR (action adj plans) OR (law OR laws) OR (rule OR rules) OR (decree OR decrees) OR (decision OR decisions) OR (act OR act) OR framework OR initiative OR campaign).mp. OR (National Health Programs.mp. OR National Health Programs/) OR (evaluation.mp. OR Evaluation Studies as Topic/) OR (Feasibility Studies/ OR feasibility.mp.) OR (Outcome.mp. OR "Outcome Assessment (Health Care)"/) OR (outcomes OR output OR outputs OR impact OR impacts).mp. OR (barriers and facilitators).mp.) AND ((Government Publications as Topic/ OR Government Programs/ OR Government/ OR Local Government/ OR Government Publications/ OR Government.mp.) OR (((non-government adj organisation) OR (non-governmental adj organisation) OR (non-government adj organization) OR (non-governmental adj organization) OR (local adj authority) OR (local adj authorities) OR authority OR (organisation OR organization) OR organisation OR organization).mp. OR Organizations/ OR (organisational OR organizational).mp. OR (public adj authority).mp. OR (public adj authorities).mp. OR state.mp. OR (public adj body).mp. OR (public adj bodies).mp. OR (municipality OR municipalities).mp. OR (ministry OR ministries).mp. OR (department OR departments).mp. OR arrondissement.mp. OR arrondissements.mp. OR province mp. OR provinces.mp. OR ministry.mp.) OR (Voluntary Health Agencies/ OR agency mp. OR agencies.mp. OR (regional adj office).mp. OR (regional adj offices).mp. OR (region OR regional).mp. OR (county adj councils).mp. OR (county adj council).mp. OR (regional adj health adj authorities).mp. OR (regional adj health adj authority).mp. OR (regional adj health adj department).mp. OR (regional adj health adj departments).mp. OR (local adj government).mp. OR voluntary.mp. OR (charity OR charities).mp.)) AND (((Austria OR Austrian OR Belgium OR Belgian OR Belge OR Bosnia OR Britain OR British OR United Kingdom OR (United adj kingdom) OR England OR Scotland OR Scottish OR Alba OR Wales OR Welsh OR Cymru OR (Northern adj Ireland) OR Bulgaria OR Bulgarian OR Croatia OR Croatian OR Cyprus OR Cyprian OR Czech OR (Czech adj Republic) OR Denmark OR Danish OR Estonia OR Estonian OR Finland OR Finnish OR France OR French OR German OR Germany OR Greek OR Greece OR Hungary OR Hungarian OR Ireland OR Irish OR Italy OR Italian OR Latvia OR Latvian OR Lithuania OR Lithuanian OR Luxembourg OR Luxembourgian OR Malta OR Maltese OR Netherlands OR Dutch OR Holland OR Poland OR Polish OR Portugal OR Portuguese OR Romanian OR Romanian OR Slovakian OR Slovak OR Slovenia OR Slovenian OR Spain OR Spanish OR Sweden OR Swedish).mp.) Limit to yr="2013-Current") OR ((Albania OR Albanian OR Andorra OR Andorran OR Armenia OR Armenian OR Azerbaijan OR Azerbaijani OR Belarus OR Belarusian OR Bosnian OR (Bosnia adj Herzegovina) OR Georgian OR Georgia OR Iceland OR Icelandic

OR Israel OR Israeli OR Kazakhstan OR Kazakhstani OR Kyrgyzstan OR Kyrgyz OR Kirghiz OR Macedonian OR Macedonia OR Yugoslav OR (Former adj Yugoslav adj Republic adj of adj Macedonia) OR Monaco OR Monacan OR Montenegro OR Montenegrin OR Norway OR Norwegian OR Moldova OR Moldovan OR (Republic adj of adj Moldova) OR Russia OR Russian OR (San adj Marino) OR Sammarinese OR Serbia OR Serbian OR Switzerland OR Swiss OR Tajikistan OR Tajik OR Tadzhik OR Turkey OR Turkish OR Turkmenistan OR Turkmenistani OR Ukraine OR Ukrainian OR Uzbekistan OR Uzbekistani).mp.)) Limit to yr="1995-Current") OR (World health organization.mp. OR World Health Organization/ OR WHO European Region.mp. OR European.mp. OR Europe/ OR European Union/ OR ((Eastern adj Europe) OR (Western adj Europe) OR (Southern adj Europe) OR Baltic OR (Central adj Asia) OR (Northern adj Asia) OR (Commonwealth adj of adj Independent adj States) OR CIS OR (Middle adj East) OR EU).mp.))

The following Internet search strategy (Google Chrome) was used.

((("health literacy" policy WHO EU) AND ("health literacy" + WHO) AND ("health literacy" + "European Union") AND (Literacy + "European Union") AND ("health literacy Europe" NGOs NGO "Non-governmental organisation" voluntary charity) AND ("health literacy" + EU + regional) AND ("health literacy" + EU + policy + evaluation) AND ("health literacy" +) AND ((Albania*, Andorra*, Armenia*, Austria*, Azerbaijan*, Belarus*, Belgium OR Belge OR Belgian, Bosnia* OR "Bosnia and Herzegovina", Bulgaria*, Croatia*, Cyprus OR Cypr*, Czech OR "Czech Republic", Denmark OR Danish, Estoni*, Finland OR Finn*, France OR French, Georgia, German*, Greek OR Greece, Hungar*, Iceland*, Ireland OR Irish, Israel*, Italy OR Italian*, Kazak*OR Kyrgyzstan*, Latvia*, Lithuania*, Luxembourg*, Malta OR Maltese, Monac* Montenegr*, Netherlands OR Dutch OR Holland, Norw*, Poland OR Polish, Portug*, the Republic of Moldova* OR "Republic of Moldova", Romania*, the Russian Federation, "San Marino", Serb*, Slovak*, Sloven*, Spain OR Spanish, Sweden OR Swedish, Switzerland OR Swiss, Tajik*, Macedoni*, Yugoslav, Turkey OR Turkish, Turkmenistan*, Ukrain* Britain OR British OR United Kingdom OR "United Kingdom" OR England OR Scotland OR Scottish OR Alba OR Wales OR Welsh OR Cymru OR "Northern Ireland", Uzbekistan*) Limit dates 1995–2017 for Non-EU/2013 for EU) OR "Alfabetización en salud"/"alfabetització en salut" (Spanish/Catalan) OR Spain OR Andorra OR Andalusia OR Catalonia OR Madrid OR Valencia OR Galicia OR Castile León OR Basque OR Castile-La Mancha OR "Canary Islands" OR Murcia OR Aragon OR Balearic OR Extremadura OR Asturias OR Navarre OR Cantabria OR "La Rioja") OR (Gezondheidsvaardigheden (Dutch) + Holland OR Netherlands OR Dutch) OR (Gesundheitskompetenz (German) +

Germany) OR (Alfabetizzazione sanitaria OR alfabetizzazione alla salute (Italian) + Abruzzo OR Apulia OR Puglia OR Basilicata OR Lazio OR Liguria OR Lombardy OR Lombardia OR Sardinia OR Sardegna OR Bolzano OR Veneto OR Emilia-Romagna OR Tuscany OR Toscana OR "Friuli Venezia Giulia" OR Basilicata OR Campania OR Calabria OR Molise OR Marche OR Piedmont OR Piemonte OR Umbria OR Sicily OR Sicilia OR Trentino))

The number of results for each database and website are as follows.

Bibliographic databases:
Embase [4438]
PubMed [3793]
PsycINFO [1140]
Web of Science [7143]
CINAHL [812]

Other sources:
Grey literature [15]
Expert enquiry [26]
HEALTH4EU study [7]

Selection of studies

Fig. A1.1 illustrates the selection of policies and studies based on the PRISMA statement (9).

Fig. A1.1. Selection of documents

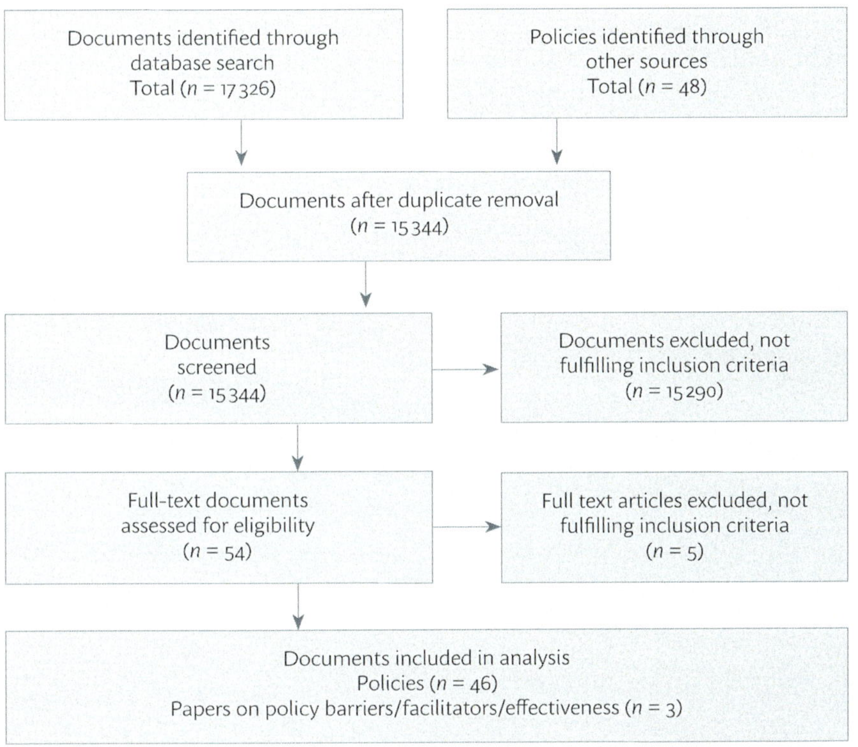

REFERENCES

1. Heijmans M, Uiters E, Rose T, Hofstede J, Devillé W, van der Heide I et al. Study on sound evidence for a better understanding of health literacy in the European Union (HEALIT4EU). Luxembourg: Publications Office of the European Union; 2015.
2. Berry J. Does health literacy matter? [blog] 19 October 2016. Leeds: NHS England; 2018 (https://www.england.nhs.uk/blog/jonathan-berry/, accessed 5 April 2018).
3. Health Literacy UK [website]. Charlton-on-Otmoor (United Kingdom): Society for Academic Primary Care; 2018 (http://www.healthliteracy.org.uk, accessed 5 April 2018).
4. Global Working Group on Health Literacy. In: International Union for Health Promotion and Education [website]. Paris: International Union for Health Promotion and Education; 2018 (http://www.iuhpe.org/index.php/en/global-working-groups-gwgs/gwg-on-health-literacy, accessed 5 April 2018).
5. Dutch Health Literacy Alliance [website]. Utrecht: Dutch Health Literacy Alliance; 2018 (http://www.gezondheidsvaardigheden.nl/english/, accessed 5 April 2018).
6. Nordic Health Literacy Network. In: Health Literacy Europe [website]. Aarhus: Global Health Literacy Academy; 2018 (https://www.healthliteracyeurope.net/nordic-health-literacy-network, accessed 5 April 2018).
7. European Network of Health Promoting Schools: the alliance of education and health: Copenhagen: WHO Regional Office for Europe; 2018 (http://www.euro.who.int/en/health-topics/Life-stages/child-and-adolescent-health/publications/Pre-2005/european-network-of-health-promoting-schools-the-alliance-of-education-and-health, accessed 14 March 2018).
8. European Health Information Initiative action network on measuring health literacy (http://www.uzg.cz/doc/Minutes-M-POHL.pdf, accessed 17 April 2018).
9. Mohr D, Liberati A, Tetzlaff J, Altman DG. Preferred reporting items for systematic reviews and meta-analyses: the PRISMA statement. Ann Intern Med. 2009;151(4):264–9.